QUIET *the* MIND

An illustrated guide on how to meditate

Written and Illustrated by Matthew Johnstone

First published in Australia in 2011 by Pan Macmillan Australia Pty Ltd
St Martins Tower, 31 Market Street, Sydney

First published in Great Britain in 2012 by Robinson

Text and illustration copyright © Matthew Johnstone 2011

5 7 9 10 8 6 4

A CIP catalogue record for this book
is available from the British Library.

ISBN 978-1-78033-118-8

Designed by Matthew Johnstone

Printed and bound in Italy by Rotolito Lombarda

Robinson
An imprint of
Little, Brown Book Group
Carmelite House
50 Victoria Embankment
London EC4Y 0DZ

An Hachette UK Company
www.hachette.co.uk

www.littlebrown.co.uk

QUIET *the* MIND

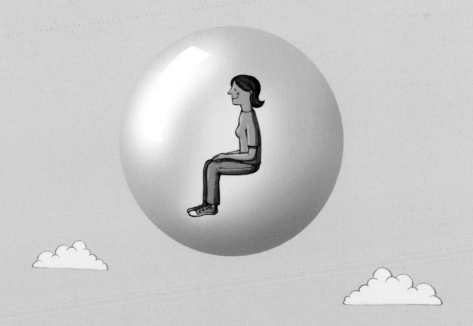

'A HEALTHY MIND HAS AN EASY BREATH.'

ANON

Foreword

You would think sitting quietly for 10–20 minutes a day would be relatively easy but for some it can be challenging,
verging on impossible. There's always something to do; somewhere to be. We're perpetually moving and bouncing around.
You can't have constant movement without constant thought, and constant thought can become exhausting.
It can bring about stress, insomnia, anxiety and depression, if left unchecked.

Modern society has made sitting still even more difficult with its tempting mantra of always 'being connected'. Cable TV, the
internet, smart phones, social networking, twittering, blogging, email, texting – all profound and useful breakthroughs in
technology but they have gobbled up our every waking moment with the need to be doing or saying something. And then
you have your day-to-day life on top of that.

With no downtime we begin to lose the precious abilities to imagine and be creative.

It's true that for our brains to be healthy they need to be flexed but it's equally important that our brains have downtime
or a regular breather. Meditation is simply a way to give our conscious brains a well-deserved break. If you learn to meditate,
your whole being will thank you for it. You will feel more 'in the present', more youthful, more energised, have greater concentration,
better moods and you will sleep more soundly. Overall you'll be better equipped and be more resilient to live this 'modern' life.

A lot of people think that meditation is an indulgence or a waste of time. There may be the fear that it could soften your drive but
in fact the opposite is true. Meditation opens up time and clears the clutter to make room for creativity and productivity.

For some people meditation has a somewhat hippy, spiritual, fringy reputation. I am by no means a meditation guru
or spiritual teacher. I've never been to an ashram, I couldn't tell you which chakra is which, I can't recite Sanskrit and I can't sit for
hours in a lotus position on a hard floor. I don't know what the meaning of life is BUT what I do know is that life is so much better
when I meditate. There are many forms of meditation that all have their differing benefits, subtleties and techniques; the message and
visual concepts in this book are simply about sitting with intention while bringing focus and mindfulness to our breath.

I suggest reading through this book a couple of times before beginning a meditation practice, just so the visual concepts have
time to sink in. Most importantly, try to bring attention to your breath while you're going through it. Every time you see the words
'in and out' consciously become aware of your breathing and, when you do, consciously allow yourself to relax and to feel calm.

Matthew Johnstone

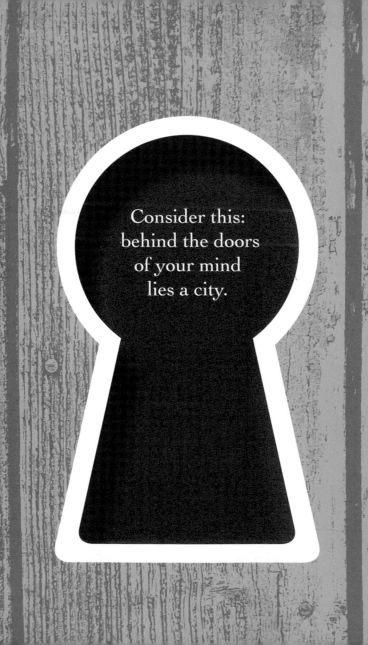

Consider this:
behind the doors
of your mind
lies a city.

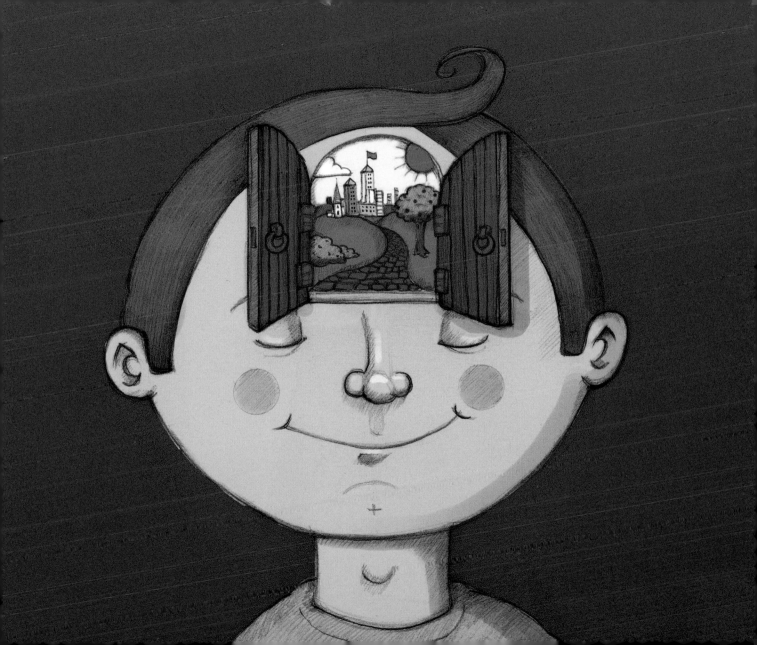

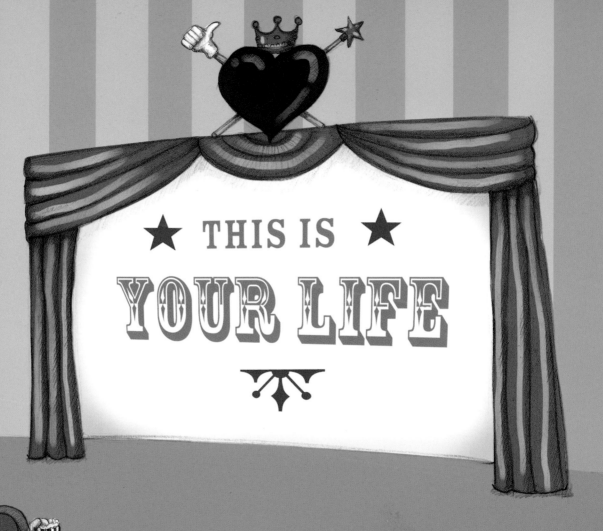

★ THIS IS ★

YOUR LIFE

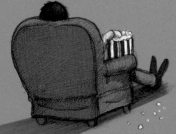

Where you'll find cinemas just for you.

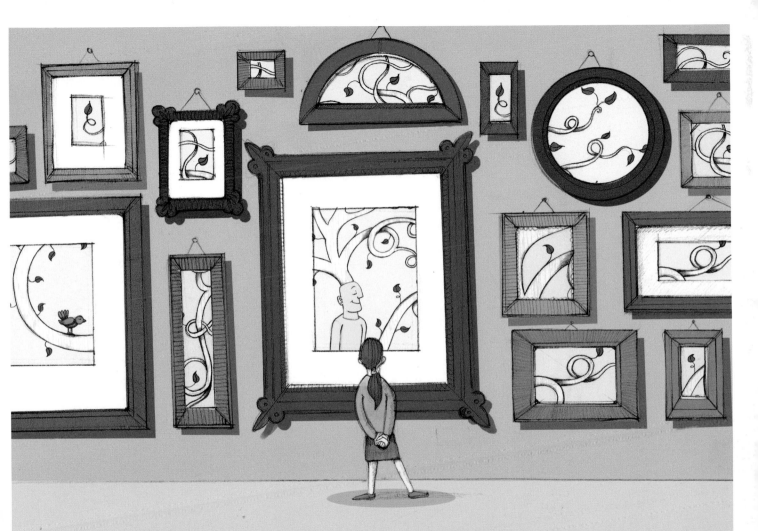

Art galleries that are always open for inspiration.

170-864

AUTHOR	Your Goodself
TITLE	A Moment of Clarity

DATE DUE	BORROWER'S NAME

Y
G

Libraries full of
memories and future
plans.

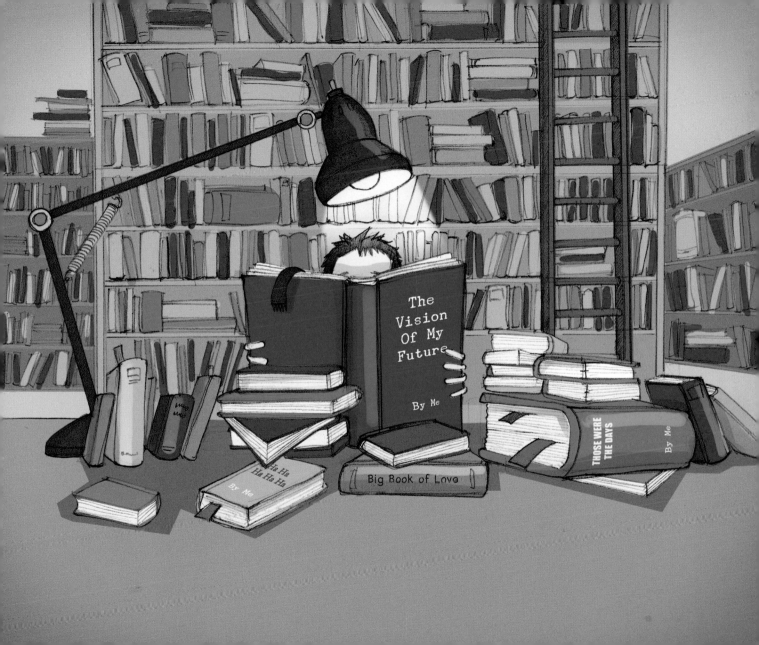

There are parks where the mind can roam free.

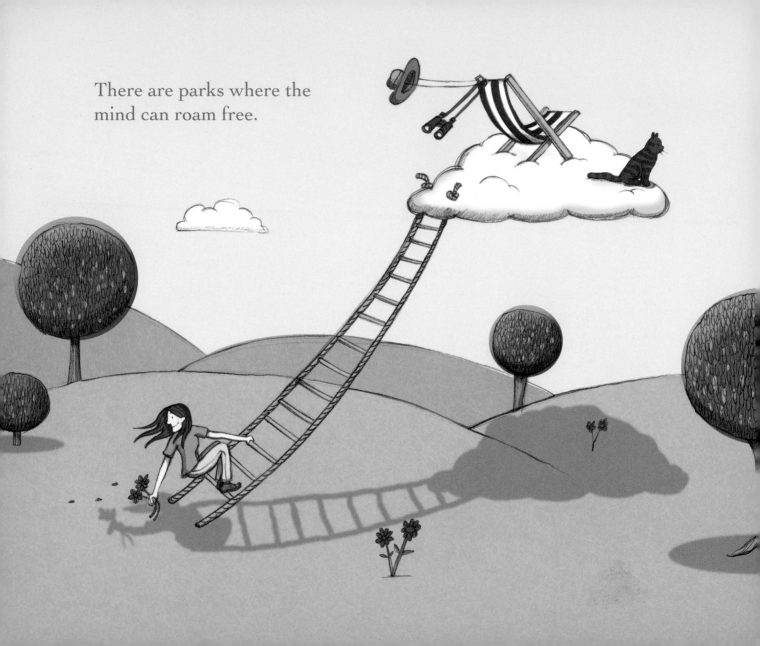

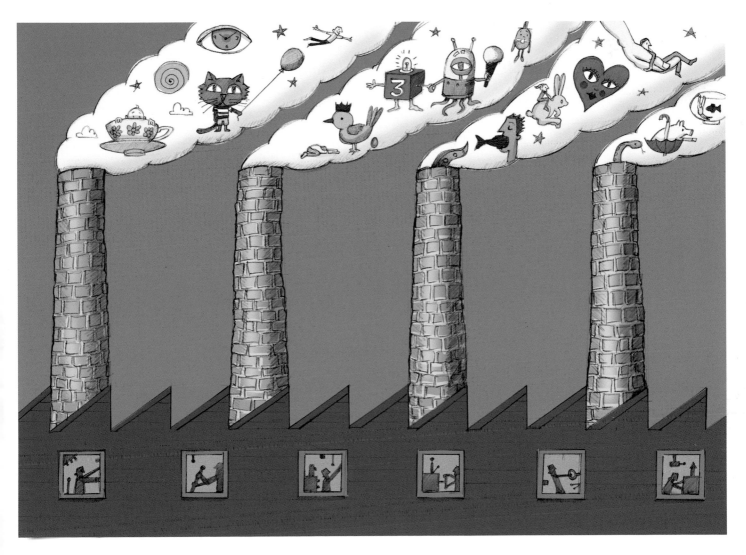

Vast factories where dreams and creativity are made.

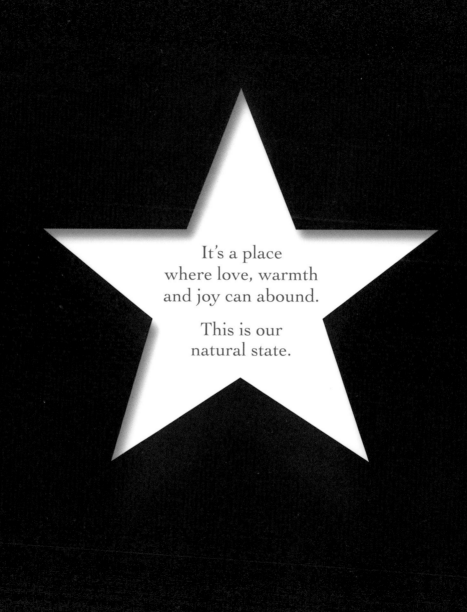

It's a place
where love, warmth
and joy can abound.

This is our
natural state.

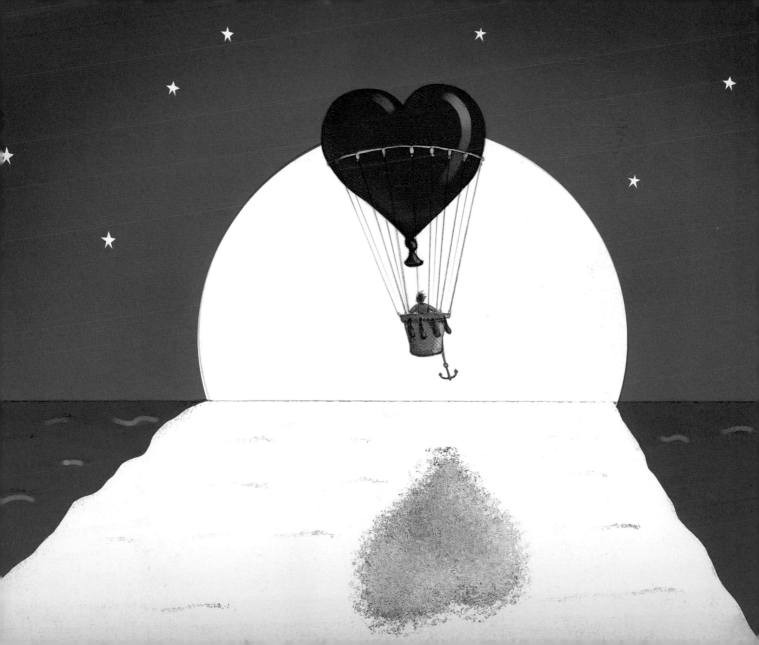

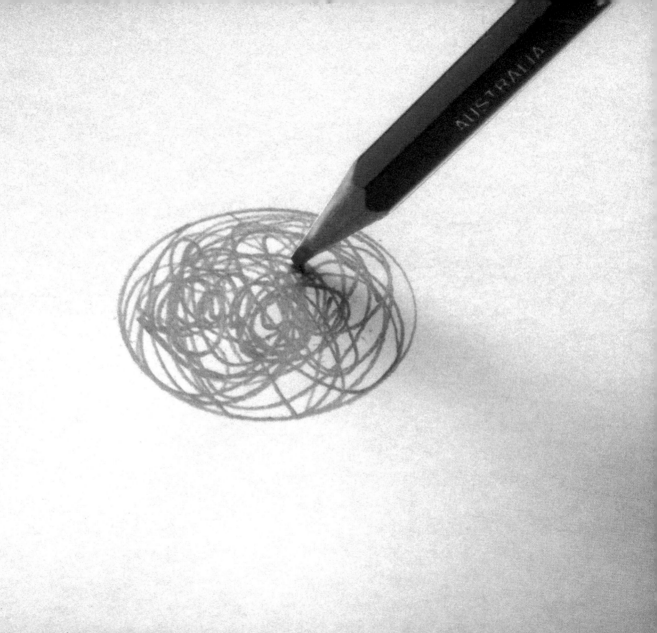

Sadly the landscape of our mind doesn't always stay so pristine – it can become polluted with a negative style of thinking.

Here's where it can go awry and why it's so important to learn how to *quiet the mind*.

24/7

Over a 24-hour period we can process up to 70,000 thoughts and this continues even as we sleep. Each day contains 86,400 seconds so that equates to a different thought every 1.2 seconds or two thoughts for every heartbeat.

Basically the brain never shuts up!

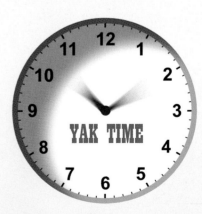

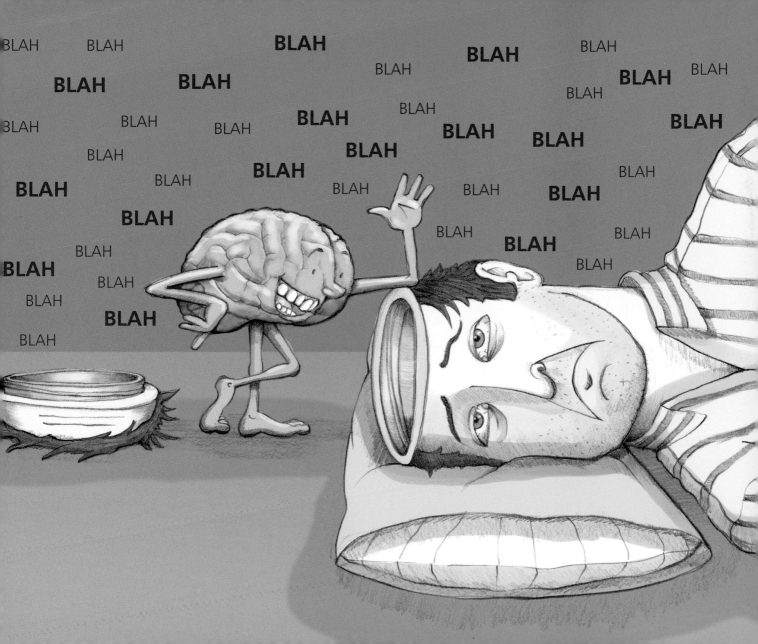

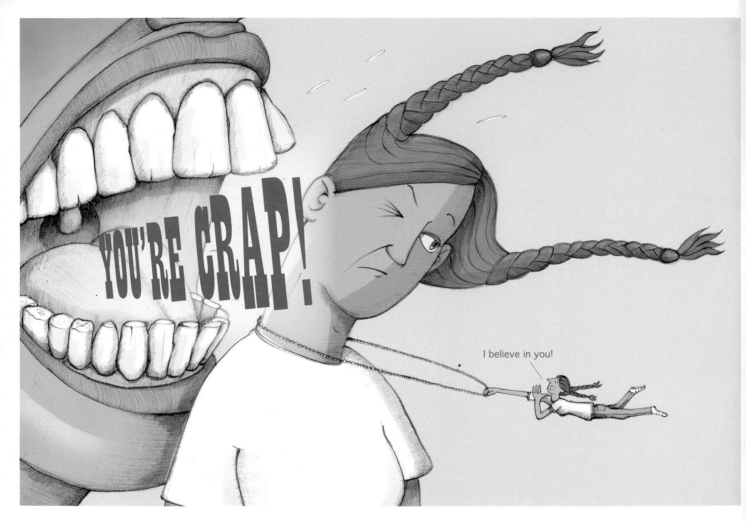

A lot of our thoughts are the eternal internal dialogue, which, if left unchecked, can turn to the dark side. This negative kind of thinking can become much more persuasive and dominant than the positive and supportive kind.

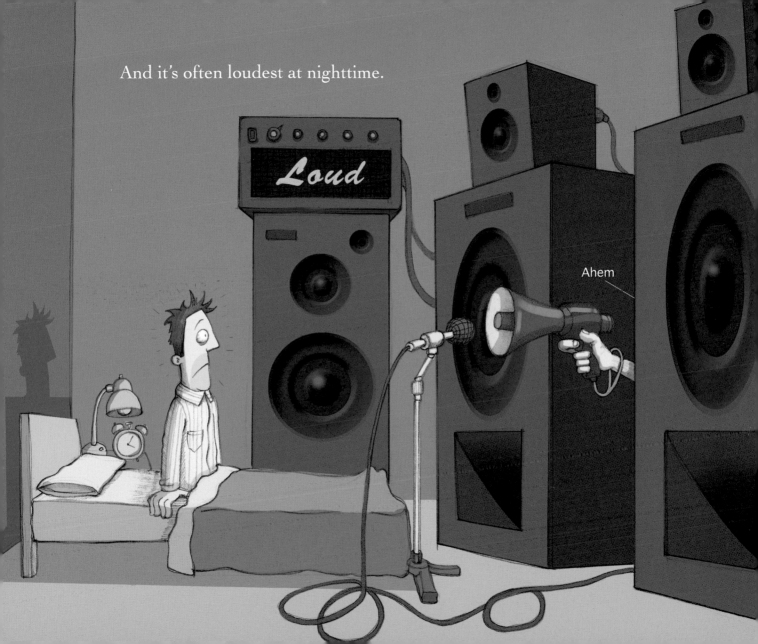

Thoughts can become obsessive
and intrusive; they can also become
stuck and repetitive.

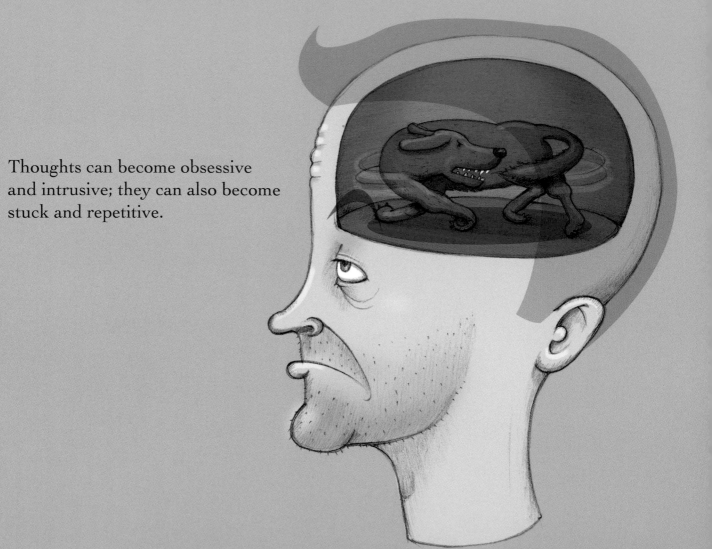

This is because within our mental library there is a huge section dedicated solely to complaints, woes, fears, regrets and hurts.

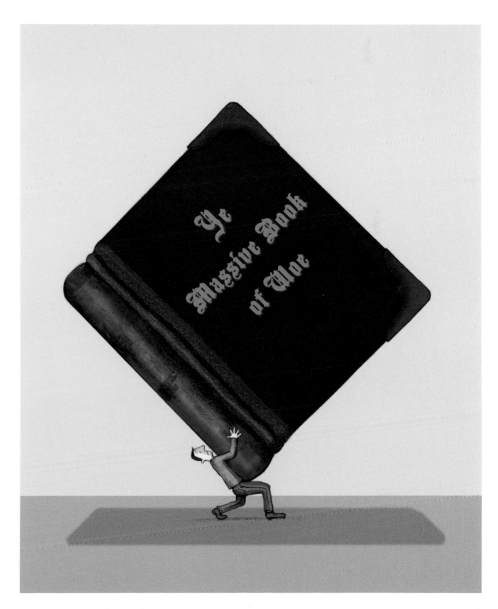

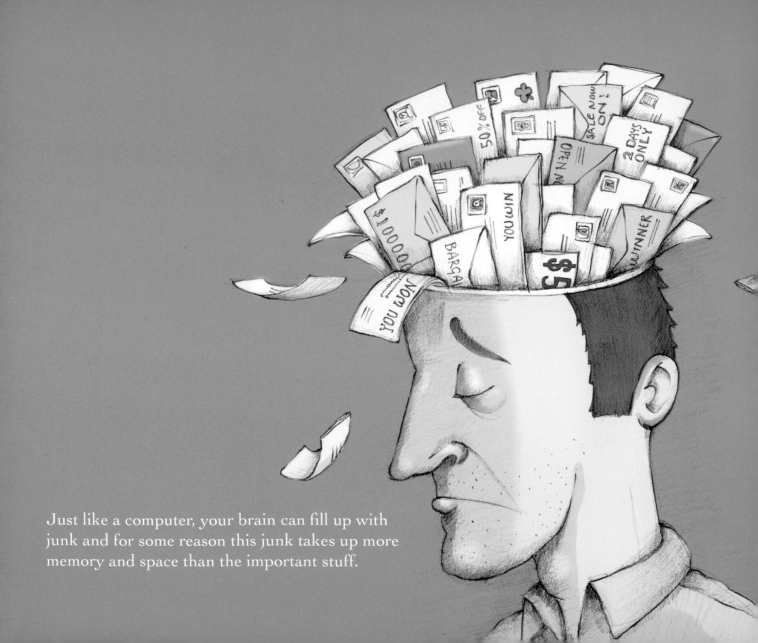

Just like a computer, your brain can fill up with junk and for some reason this junk takes up more memory and space than the important stuff.

If your memory is full of junk it becomes difficult to concentrate.

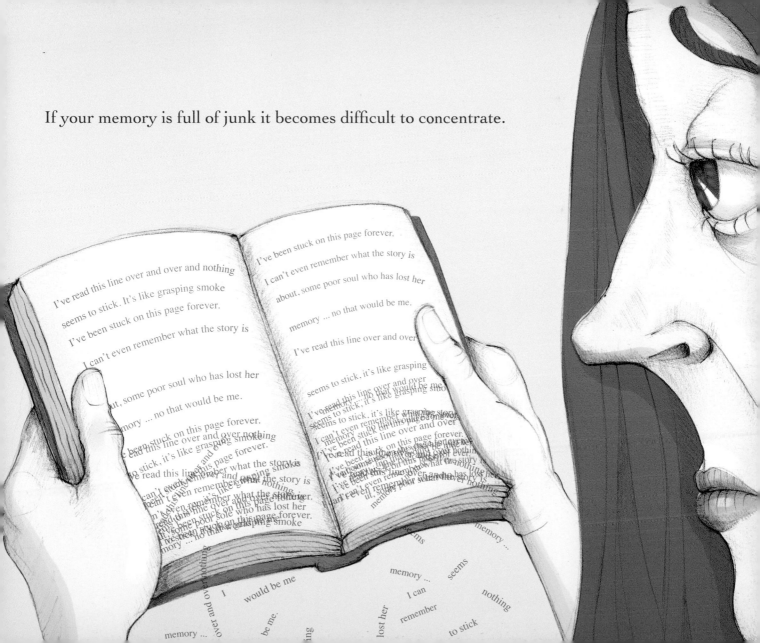

Recalling information can be like trying to pick up marbles on a rolling ship.

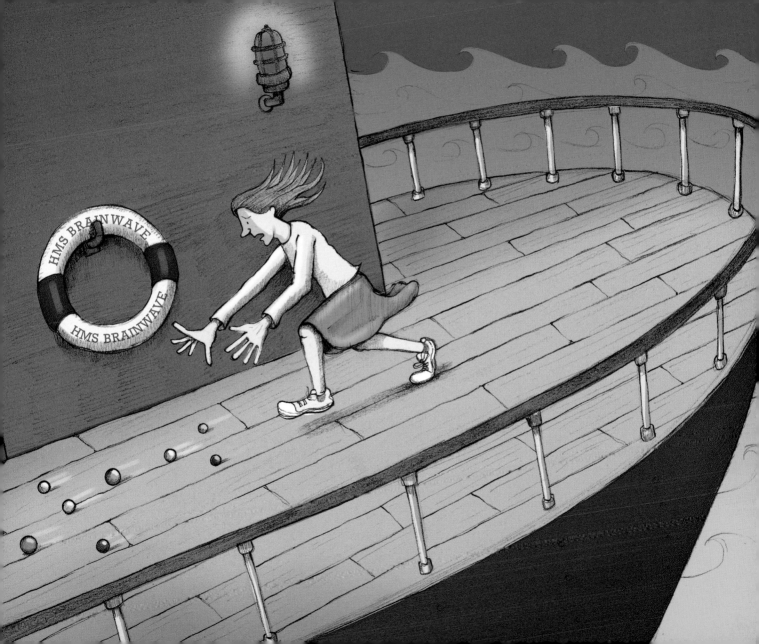

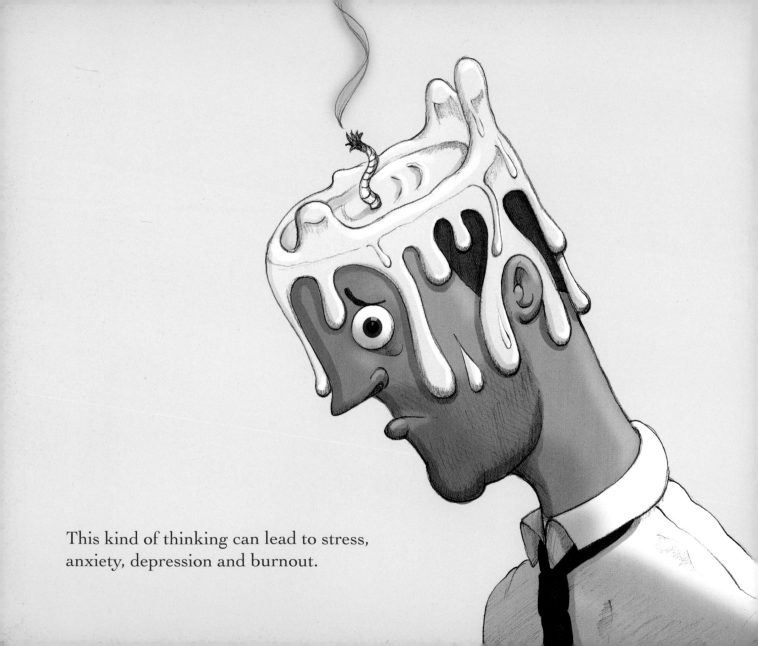

This kind of thinking can lead to stress,
anxiety, depression and burnout.

There is a simple solution that can make you calmer, more focused, more present and happier.

It has been proven to reduce stress, improve metabolism, reduce pain, lower blood pressure, improve respiration and enhance brain function.

It costs nothing and all you have to do is

NOTHING.

Here's how.

WHEN

Meditation when done correctly can be more restorative than sleep.
Any time is a great time to meditate but one of the best times is half an hour
before you typically get up as it is the quietest time of the day. Don't try
to meditate while you're still lying in bed; it's not nearly as effective.

Late afternoon or early evening are the other optimal times.
Some find meditating before bedtime helpful for a good night's sleep.

If you're waking in the night and can't get back to sleep,
it can be more beneficial to physically get up and
meditate rather than wasting precious energy tossing
and turning. Once you've calmed your thoughts
down, you may find getting back to sleep a lot easier.

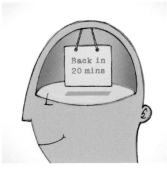

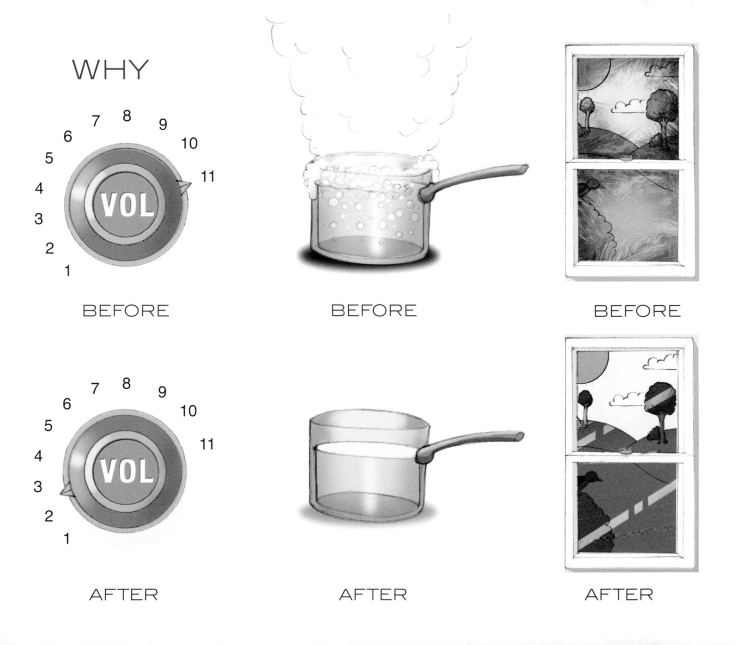

WHY

BEFORE   BEFORE   BEFORE

AFTER   AFTER   AFTER

PREPARATION

For best results it's important to 'hush proof' your surroundings.

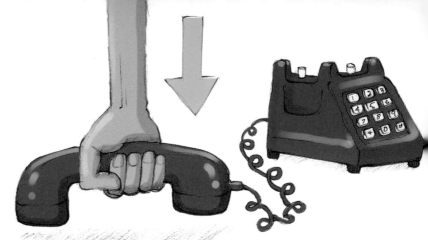

Off the hook.

'It's SHHHH time.'

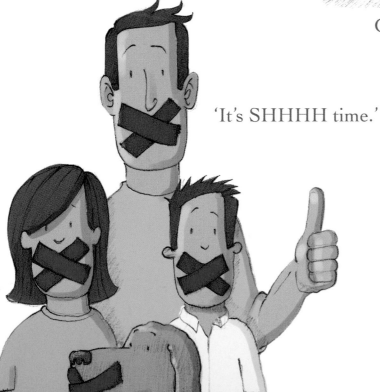

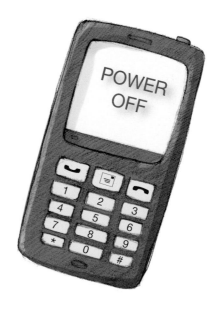

EQUIPMENT

A firm but comfortable upright chair.

Although not mandatory, a pair of earplugs or noise-cancelling headphones can minimise noise and bring more attention to the breath.

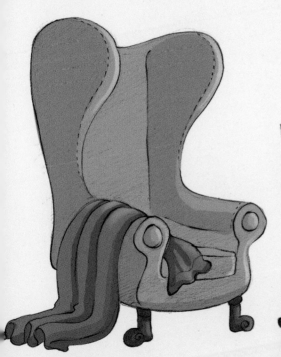

If need be, a blanket to keep warm.

A reminder to keep the peace.

QUIET PLEASE

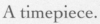

A timepiece.

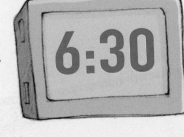

6:30

A cushion to place behind your lower back. This helps maintain an upright posture.

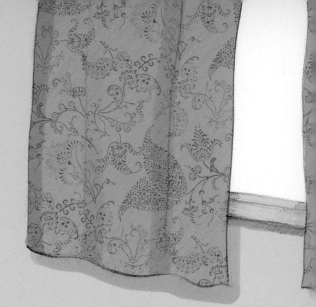

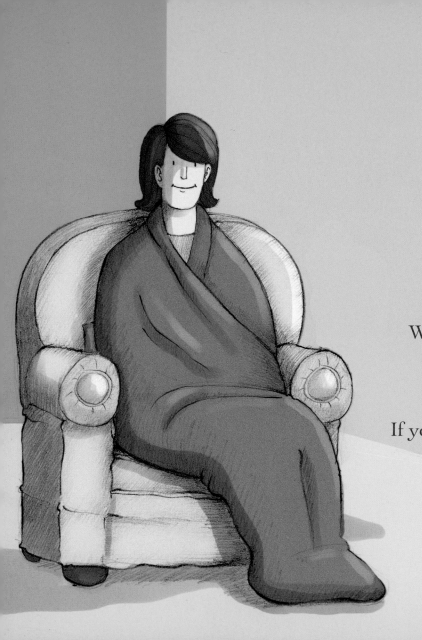

When meditating use the quietest room
in the house. Make the space as snug,
peaceful and comfortable as possible.

If you meditate in total darkness you may
nod off so use a soft, ambient light.

THE POSTURE

Your posture should be as upright and symmetrical as possible.

Think of yourself as a guard at Buckingham Palace, only sitting down.

This posture is alert, but relaxed.

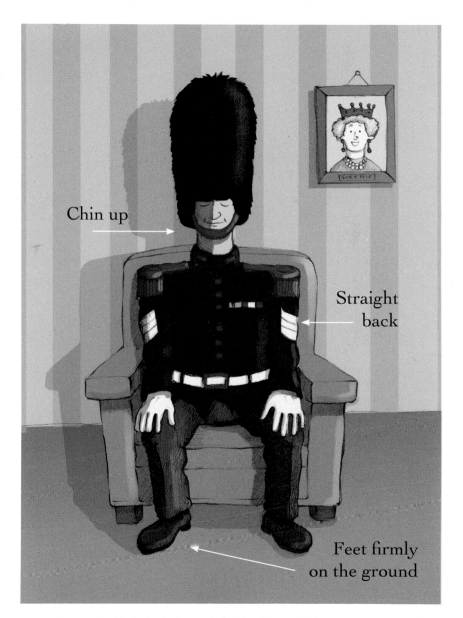

Chin up

Straight back

Feet firmly on the ground

TO WRINKLE AND TO UNWRINKLE

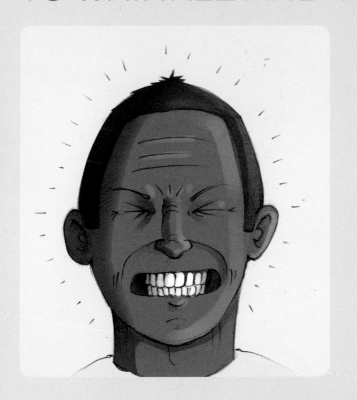 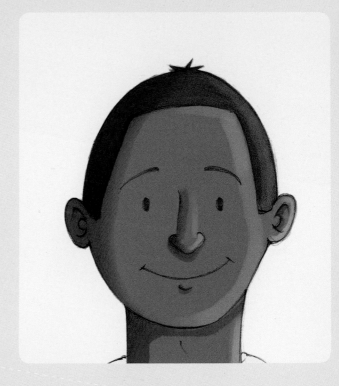

Before you do anything, you could use the following technique to help your body relax. Starting with your feet and toes gently tense and relax those muscles and slowly work your way up through your body to the top of your head. Feel the contrast between the muscles when they are tense and when they are relaxed. This brings an awareness or an 'awaken-ness' to our bodies.

WHAT TO DO WITH YOUR HANDS

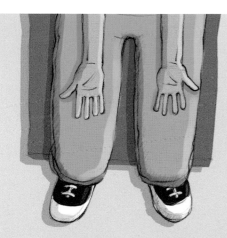 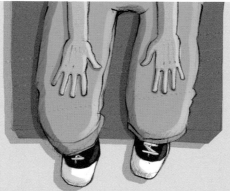 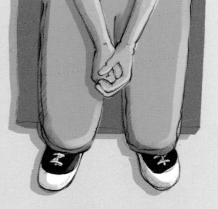

Place palms up.

Or palms down, whichever is more comfortable.

Or place one hand comfortably in the other.

Think of a cat curled up in a basket.

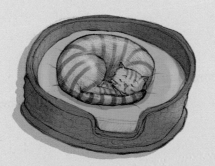

THE MAKING OF A BLANK CANVAS

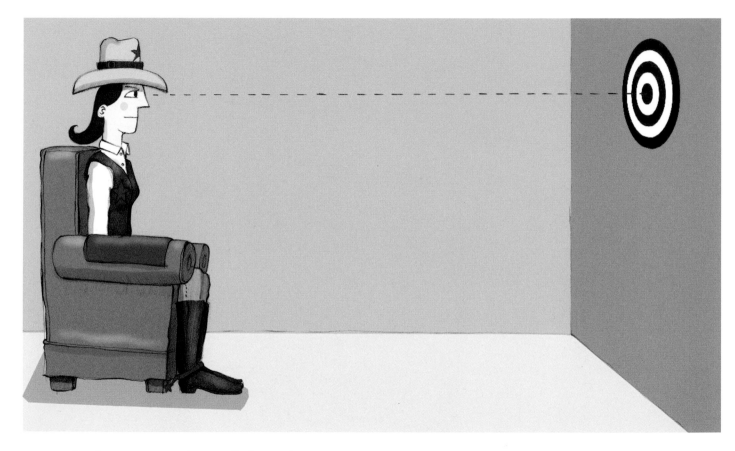

Next, find a spot on the wall directly in front of you and give it the 1000-yard stare. This is a time to begin turning down the internal dialogue. Take 3 to 6 deep, slow breaths. Soften your focus and then slowly close your eyes.

COME WITHIN

While you keep your eyes shut, focus on the sounds outside the room. You might hear cars, a dog barking, the wind. Acknowledge these sounds.

Next, bring your focus to the sounds within the room. You may hear a clock, the hum of an electrical appliance, the house creaking. Acknowledge these sounds, too.

Now listen to the sounds within your body, your breath, your heartbeat, the faint ringing in your ears. This is where you want your attention to be; within yourself, not outside it.

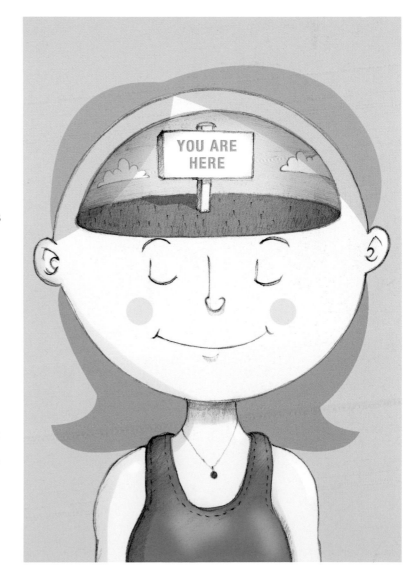

THE NOSE IS WHERE IT'S AT

Although this book offers many visual analogies to consider, the most important
thing to remember in meditation is your nose and the breath that flows in and out of it.

Think of your nose as a lighthouse from which you take all your meditative bearings.

If you get lost in a sea of thought, think of your lighthouse and come back to your breath.

If you hear a dog bark, come back to your breath.

If you feel uncomfortable, move gently and come back to your breath.

Breathing in and out; nice and slow and steady.

... in and out ... in and out ... in and out ...

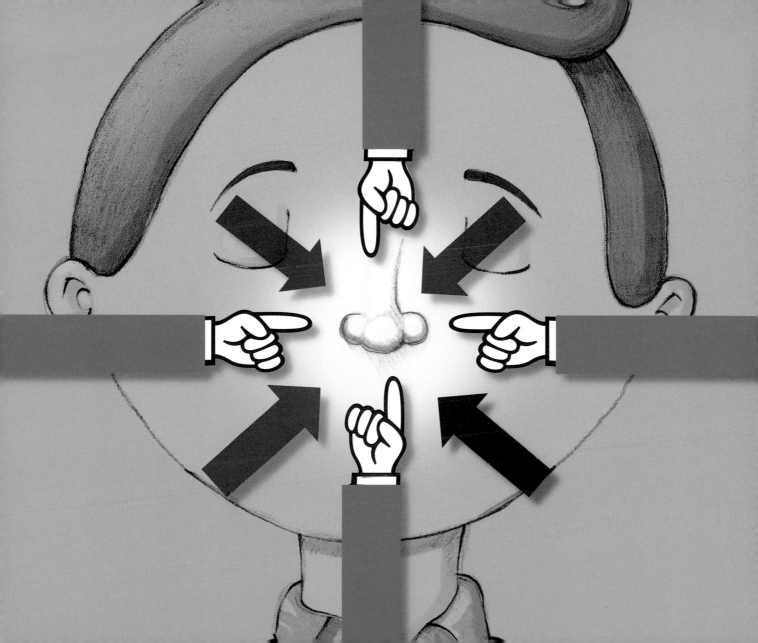

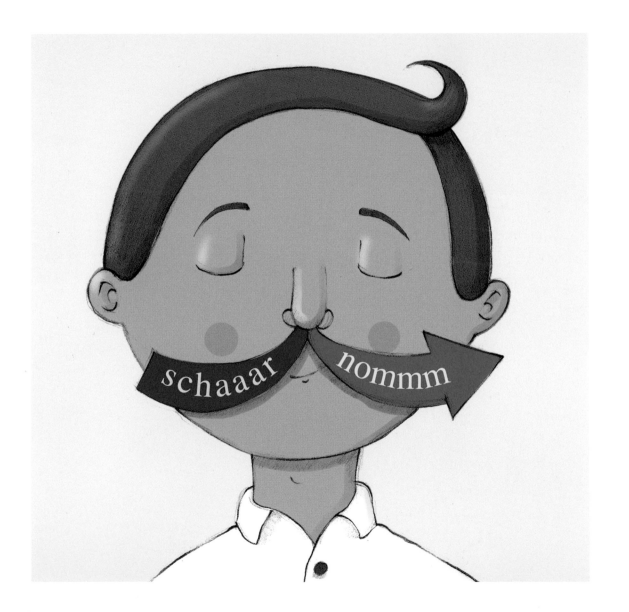

THE MANTRA MOUSTACHE

Using a word or a mantra is a useful way to focus on the breath.
It also stops the mind wandering off into a rambling wilderness.
Choose gentle, soft, rounded words. Neutral words that don't have any
particular association or raise any particular feeling.

A mantra can be two words or one word with two syllables
(one for each in and out breath).

I – Am   *Here – Now*   *Lov – ing*

Mantras can mean nothing at all; you can make up your own.

Schaaar – nommm   *Baaaar – rommm*   *Gaaar – rommm*

When using a mantra with your breath, try to become gently
aware of the space between each word, syllable and breath
– this is where stillness and silence sit.

... in and out ... in and out ... in and out ...

QUIET THOUGHTS TO KEEP IN MIND

Gently press the tip of your tongue against the roof of your mouth. This reminds us to keep our head upright. It's also another safety measure against nodding off.

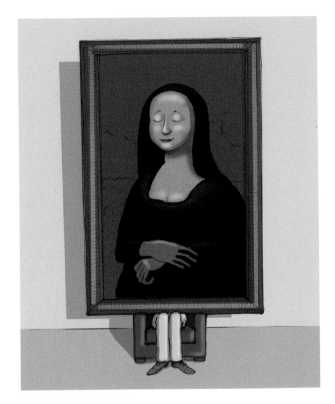

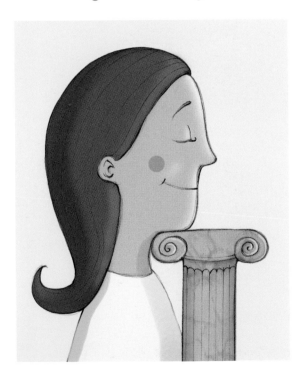

Smiling releases endorphins (the brain's natural relaxant), so picture yourself with a gentle smile and you'll probably have one during meditation.

... in and out ... in and out ... in and out ...

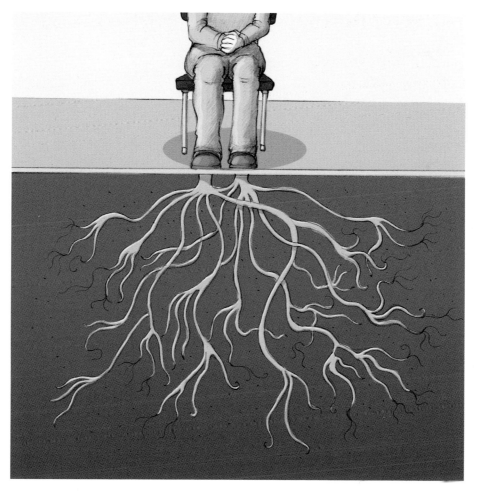

Each time you breathe in and out, think of your feet growing roots into the floor.
The deeper the roots go, the deeper the meditation.
This thought anchors you into the moment and keeps you centred.

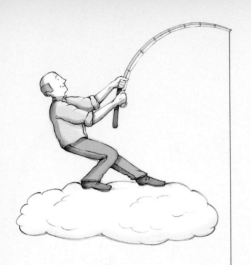

As you breathe into your meditation,
picture a little person pulling an invisible line
right up through your spine, your neck
and through the top of your head.

You are sitting with purpose.

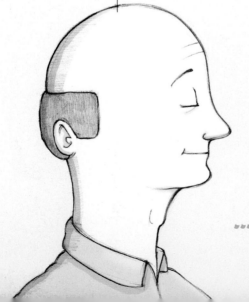

... in and out ... in and out ...

With regular meditation practice, keeping your head and posture upright becomes effortless. You will feel your spine and neck elongating.

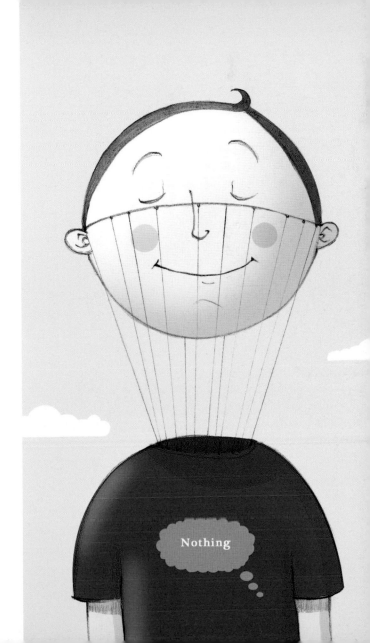

INCOMING THOUGHTS

When you meditate, especially in the beginning, thoughts will naturally bubble to the surface. These thoughts will include things you have to do, extensions of conversations, frustrations, self-criticism, planning for the future or reliving the past. Anything and everything will try to disturb your peace of mind.

The most important thing is <u>NOT</u> to get upset with yourself. Simply acknowledge these thoughts; then let them go. Do not pursue them, judge them or reject them. Thoughts during meditation can be the mind's way of releasing stress and tension; think of it as bubbles in a champagne glass. Even when a meditation is mentally turbulent, there is still great benefit in sitting quietly.

Meditation is a time to be gentle with yourself.
Don't get upset because you are having thoughts, nodding off or needing to itch.

Turning down the 'thought valve' can be tricky but with patience and
a degree of discipline it can be done.

This is why meditation is called a practice.

... in and out ... in and out ...

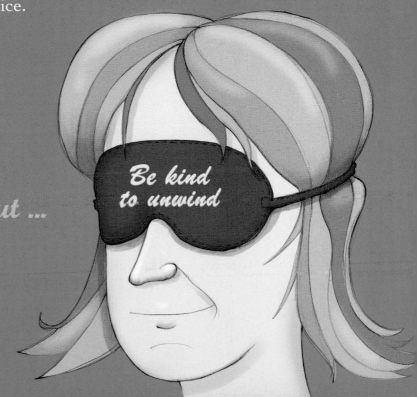

Think of your thoughts as a flock of dozing sheep;
if one makes a run for it, send out the sheepdog to gently bring it back.

... in and out ... in and out ... in and out ...

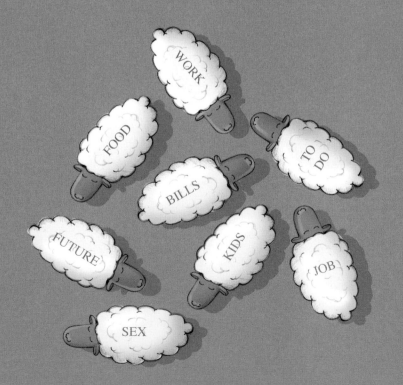

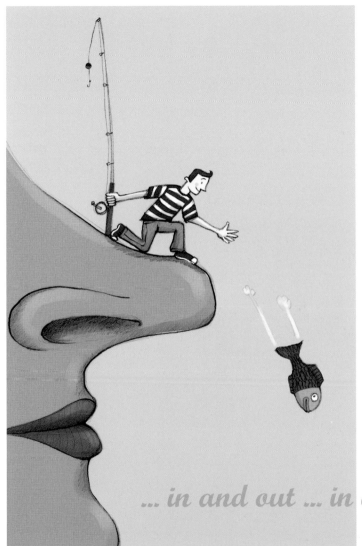

Or think of it as fishing and errant thoughts are the fish. When you catch a thought, acknowledge it then release it.

No harm done.

Back to the breath.

... in and out ... in and out ... in and out ...

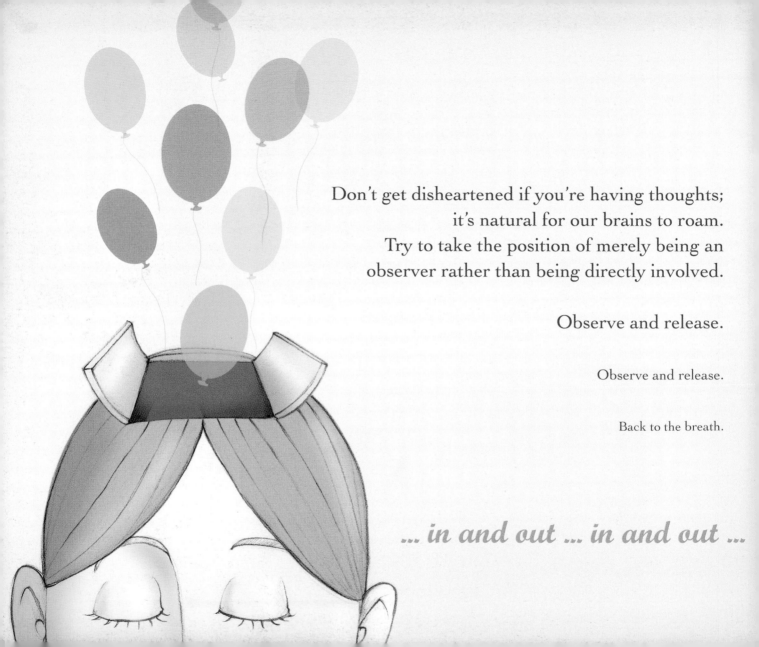

Don't get disheartened if you're having thoughts;
it's natural for our brains to roam.
Try to take the position of merely being an
observer rather than being directly involved.

Observe and release.

Observe and release.

Back to the breath.

... in and out ... in and out ...

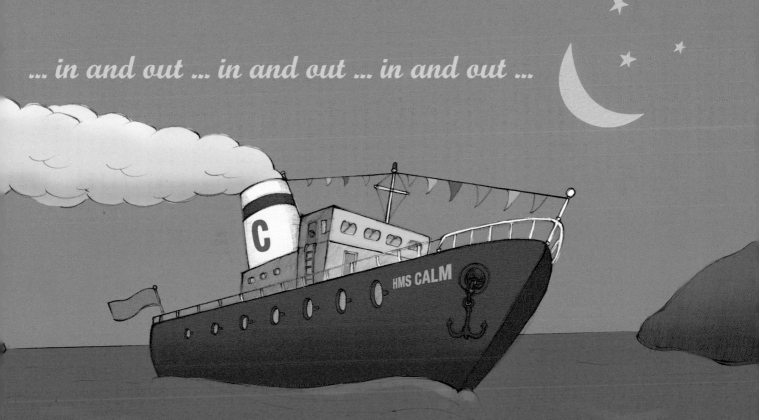

... in and out ... in and out ... in and out ...

As you breathe into your meditation, become aware of your mind and body
slowing down like a ship that has been on 'full steam ahead' through rough seas.
It slows right down as it enters the stillness of an inner harbour.

PICTURE YOURSELF

Before you begin to meditate it can be helpful to use visual imagery to help get you into the zone. The following pages have some suggestions of what to try. Obviously you can make up your own, just try not to overthink it.

Picture yourself as a scuba diver sitting on a rock.

The water is warm; it's clear and it's very tranquil.

Think of the ocean's surface as your conscious mind – it's there, it may even be a bit choppy – but it's not affecting you.

Each time you breathe out, oxygen bubbles slowly make their way to the surface.

Like the ocean around you, you become more and more still.

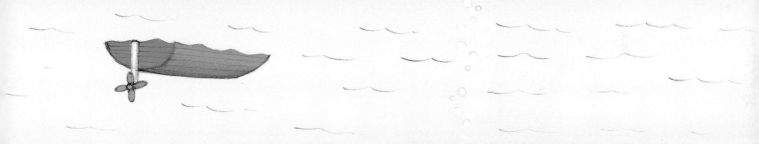

... in and out ... in and out ... in and out ...

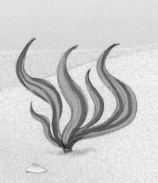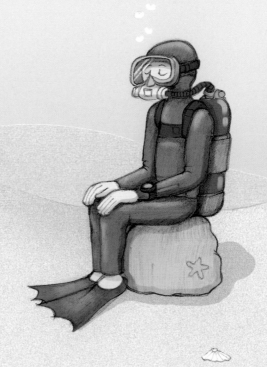

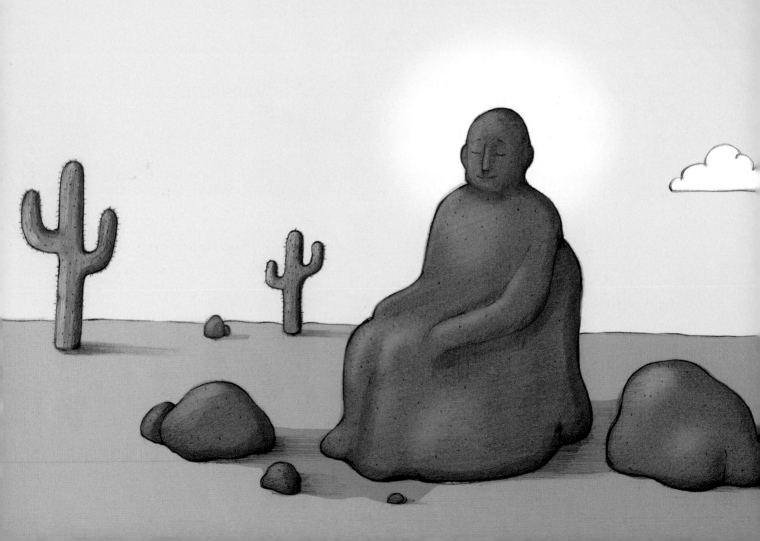

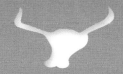

Think of yourself as a big stone sitting in peaceful permanence.
You are being warmed by the sun.

You are aware of your surroundings but nothing can bother you.

You are a warm stone that has been sitting there for thousands of years.

Observant yet not involved.

... in and out ... in and out ... in and out ...

Think of yourself in deep space.
Your reliable ship is on autopilot – little lights blink softly.
You have nothing to worry about.

Each time you breathe in and out the stars shine more brightly
and you begin to feel as expansive as the universe.

... in and out ... in and out ... in and out ...

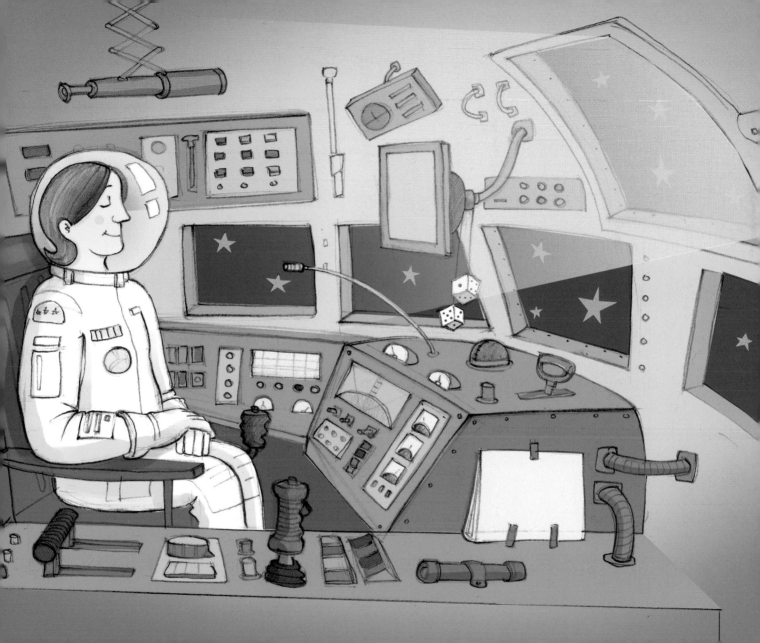

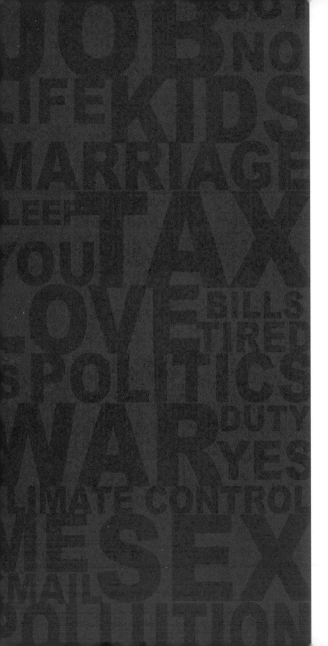

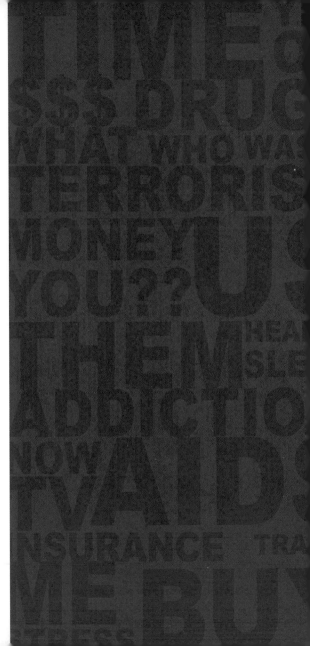

There is no
place quieter
than the
space that
exists
between
each breath.

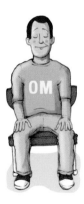

With practice you can get to a place
of incredible stillness. It's like being
in a room with nothing in it,
including yourself.

Nowhere to go. No one to see.
Nothing to do. Simply breathe.

... in and out ... in and out ... in and out ...

When meditating you may experience unusual sensations, most of which are very pleasant. Try not to focus your attention on them; rather, just go with it.

Serenity

Energy Rushes

Insight

Tingling

Slowing of
the Heart
and Breath

Feelings of
Weightlessness

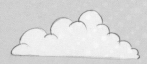

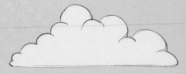

... in and out ... in and out ...

After 20 minutes or so (go longer if you want to),
gradually bring your awareness back into the room
and your body. When you're good and ready,
take a few nice, deep breaths, fill the lungs
and gently open your eyes.

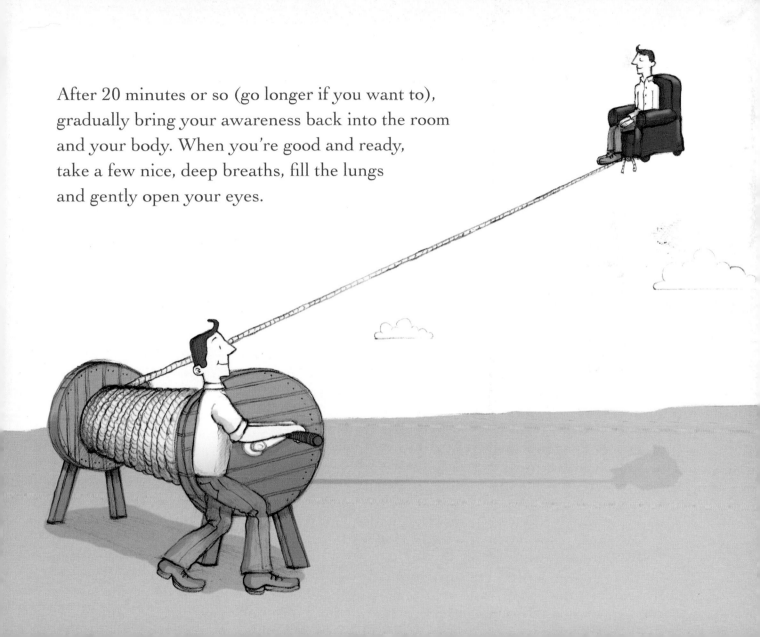

Before you get up and move about, just sit consciously for a minute
or two in silence while remaining aware of your breath.

Notice how still everything is.

Think about the day ahead or the day just been.

Think about how you wish to be around others.

Think about what you truly have to be grateful for.

Think about how peaceful you feel right in this moment – keep that peace with you.

Stand up and have a good stretch.

THE BEST MEDICATION IS **DAILY MEDITATION**

MEDITATION

Practise
twice daily
before and
after meals

FINAL ILLUMINATING THOUGHTS

This book has many visual ideas and metaphors on how to get into the meditative zone.
None of them are a 'must do!' they are simply a guide or a set of tools.

The important thing is not to overthink meditation. When you become accomplished at riding a bicycle, although you have to remain alert, compute many complex actions and judgements, you don't overthink it. When you're cycling you're not thinking, 'I must keep peddling! I must keep my balance! I must keep my hands on the handlebars!' There are only continual, subtle adjustments that result in a smooth journey. It is the same for meditation.

So do your mind, your body, your soul a big favour by committing to a practice once or twice a day, for four to six weeks. During that time, keep a journal and jot down how your meditation went, things you noticed and how you felt before and after. Hopefully you will feel the benefits, and incorporate a practice into your day-to-day life.

THINGS TO KEEP IN (A QUIET) MIND:

- **The breath is the key**
- **There are no good or bad, right or wrong ways to meditate**
- **Be kind to yourself**
- **Observe thoughts and then release**
- **A mantra makes the breath go round**
- **Do what works best for you**
- **Be proud of yourself for giving this a go**
- **Don't meditate while riding a bicycle**

Om-wards and outwards!

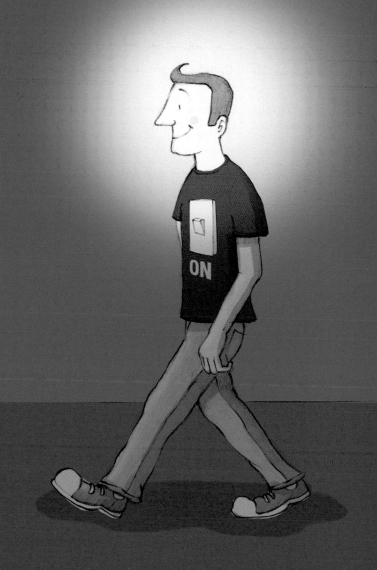

There are many books on meditation. This book is really meditation for beginners; it is for those who are curious but have never known where to start. Meditation has evolved over thousands of years; there are myriad forms of meditation and it is a part of many religions and spiritual paths.

In more recent times the mental health sector has been finding a great role for meditation and mindfulness in combating mental illnesses such as depression, anxiety, post-traumatic stress and so on.

So if you wish to take your meditation practice further or learn more about mindfulness, you could start by checking out the following books:

Kabat-Zinn, Jon (2004) *Wherever You Go, There You are: Mindfulness Meditation for Everyday Life*, Piatkus

Tolle, Eckhart (2001) *The Power of Now: A Guide to Spiritual Enlightenment*, New World Library

Thich, Hanh Nhat (1999) The Miracle of Mindfulness: An Introduction to the Practice of Meditation, Beacon Press

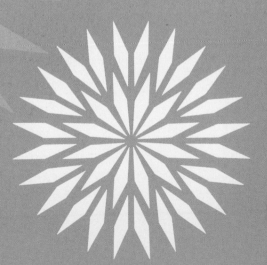